Introduction

The back can experience a variety of [injuries to the bones, ligaments,] and muscles in the area. It is one of t[he...] almost 60% to 90% of us experiencing ~~back pain within~~ our lifetime. The most common causes of lower back pain include muscle strains and arthritis. People often experience a dull ache or sharp pain, which may radiate to the gluteal (buttocks) region. At times, the pain is worsened with specific movements, including bending forward (flexion), bending backward (extension), or rotating to the side. Other times, the pain is worse upon awakening in the morning and is associated with stiffness, as in arthritis. More severe pain may be due to a variety of other causes, including a fracture from trauma or a disc herniation. Such pain may be associated with numbness in the lower leg or exacerbation with coughing/sneezing. People experiencing such symptoms should seek further evaluation.

Fortunately, the causes of most acute lower back pain are not serious and will improve over a relatively short period of time. Most symptoms may be treated over a several-week period with relative rest, medication, proper stretching, and improved posture. Subsequent symptoms may be prevented by continued stretching and strengthening of the back muscles. The goal of this booklet is to describe the common causes of acute back pain relating to muscle strains, and strategies for the prevention and treatment of such injuries.

Structure (Anatomy) of the Back

The back is made up of bones, ligaments, and muscles that connect the torso to the lower body. The lower back or lumbar spine is composed of five vertebrae, which are stacked one on top of another. In between these vertebrae are discs that provide cushioning to assist with bending and turning of the lower back region. Ligaments around the vertebrae act like guide wires to allow movement of the back in multiple directions. Finally, the

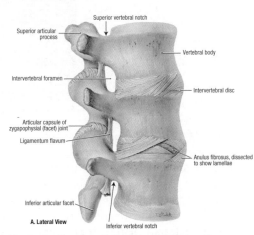

Figure 1. Drawing of the side view (lateral) lumbar spine.

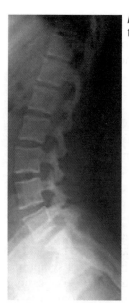

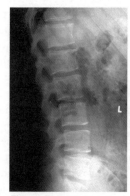

Figure 2. Lateral x-ray of the cervical spine.

Figure 3. Lateral x-ray with straight lumbar spine.

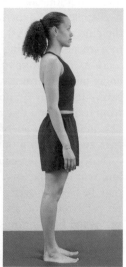

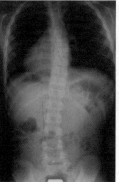

Figure 4. Lumbar spine x-ray with scoliosis.

Figure 5a. Good posture.

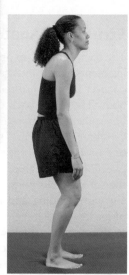

multiple layers of muscles provide additional support with motion. All of the structures protect the spinal cord, which travels down the lumbar spine sending nerves to the lower extremities. In the normal standing position, the lumbar vertebrae are slightly curved in a reverse "C" shape as shown in Figure 2. With injury, the lumbar spine may straighten due to an underlying fracture or muscle spasm (Fig. 3). Excessive curvature or scoliosis of the lumbar spine may occur with other injuries or naturally to the spine (Fig. 4). Proper posture of the lower back may help with preventing subsequent injury (Fig. 5).

Figure 5b. Poor spine posture.

Common Injuries and Disease of the Back

Fortunately, the majority of injuries to the back are due to muscle strains. Often these injuries are due to non-traumatic mechanisms that may occur due to performing an unfamiliar exercise or holding your back in an unnatural position. However, any back pain that occurs due to trauma should be evaluated by a physician to assure there is no underlying fracture. In addition, back pain associated with tingling in the lower leg should be evaluated by a physician. The following are common causes of back pain.

Acute Muscle Strain

Muscle strains are a very common cause of acute lower back pain. The pain is described as achy to sharp in nature, involving the muscles around the back, but not along the middle of the back. Often, the pain is worsened by bending forward or to the side, stretching the involved muscle. Although the pain may radiate to the gluteal region, it is not usually associated with tingling involving the lower leg. Coughing or sneezing does not typically worsen the pain. Pushing on the muscles of the lower back and stretching of the muscle will reproduce the pain. Acute lower back muscle strains will usually resolve over a 6-week period with relative rest, avoidance of activity that exacerbates the symptoms, cold or head packs, medication, and/or massage.

Disc Herniation

Back or lumbar disc herniations are less common-but more serious-injuries to the back. A disc herniation occurs when the inner substance of the disc ruptures, causing inflammation and compression of the nerves of the back. (Picture jelly coming out of a jelly donut [Fig. 6].) A disc hernation may occur when performing lifting activities or turning your head with the back flexed. Patients typically complain of sharp pain involving the region of the back with radiation of the pain to the lower leg. They may note tingling involving the thigh, leg,

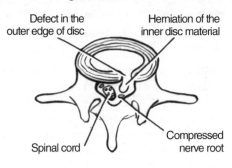

Figure 6. Lumbar disc herniation.

or foot in a specific area. The symptoms are worsened with bending forward and/or rotating to the same side. Coughing or sneezing will often make the symptoms worsen. Anyone experiencing a potential disc hernation should seek a proper evaluation by a physician. Treatment can range from the use of medication and physical therapy to surgery, depending upon the extent of the symptoms.

Arthritis

Many of us get arthritis of the spine over time. However, not everyone has pain related to arthritis of the back. Pain due to arthritis of the spine is gradual in onset, slowly occurring over weeks or months. The pain is described as dull in nature and worsened with any movement of the back. The pain may radiate toward the gluteal region, but is not associated with tingling in the lower leg. Often, patients report back stiffness upon arising in the morning and lessening of the pain during the day with continued motion. Treatments include activity modification, medication, and exercise.

Preventive Measures

As noted before, a back strain may occur due to performing an unfamiliar exercise or holding the back in an unnatural position. Common positions or deficits that can lead to subsequent back strain include:

1. Poor abdominal and lumbar spine muscle strength: Proper strength of these muscles is essential to possibly preventing subsequent injury. Strength of these "core" muscles will protect the spine when it is in an unusual or awkward position.
2. Bending forward while lifting a heavy object off the ground may place an unusual stress on the back. People usually experience a disc herniation while bending forward with rotation.
3. Holding the back rotated or twisted for a prolonged period of time.

Patients may find themselves in any of these positions during common daily activities. Any task in which the back is flexed and bent over a work-such as working at a desk or on a computer, or lifting a heavy object-may cause strain to the back muscles. Even resting can cause back strain if it is done in an improper position and too often. Finally, other associated factors contributing to possible back pain include smoking, depression, anxiety, poor job satisfaction, and lack of aerobic conditioning.

Figures 7 through 24 illustrate unnatural body positions that are common causes of back strains during everyday activities. In addition, the figures note the proper positions to help prevent such injury. The patient should consider a "work-site evaluation" to assure the proper placement of your work needs, such as your computer, to help prevent subsequent injury.

Tips:
- Keep your back straight while sitting in a chair (Figs. 7 and 8).
- Use a chair with proper support of the back, shoulders, and arms to prevent your head being thrust forward and your back being curved for a prolonged period of time (Figs. 9 and 10).

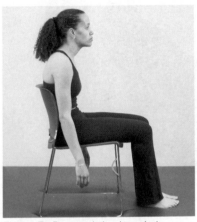

Figure 7. Person sitting in a chair, slouched forward.

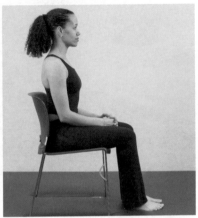

Figure 8. Person sitting in a chair with correct posture.

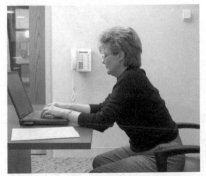

Figure 9. Person working on a desk leaning forward.

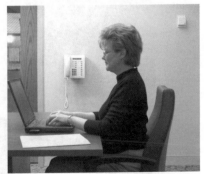

Figure 10. Person working on a desk with proper posture and chair support.

- Make sure your chair is the right height, neither too low nor too high. Sit straight and avoid having to twist or stretch forward while working, eating, and so forth (Figs. 11 and 12).

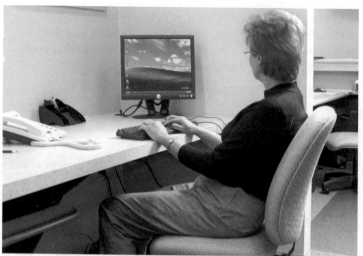

Figure 11. Person at the desk slouching and rotated while typing on a computer.

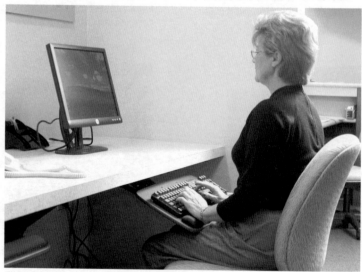

Figure 12. Person with proper alignment of work site to type on a computer.

- Make sure your car seat is adjusted properly. If it is too far forward, you will need to stretch your back forward to see (Figs. 13 and 14).

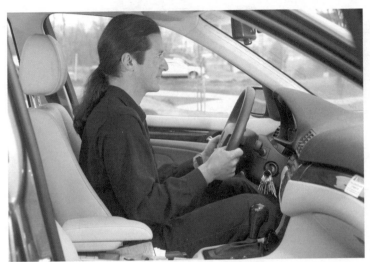

Figure 13. Person driving in car with incorrect posture.

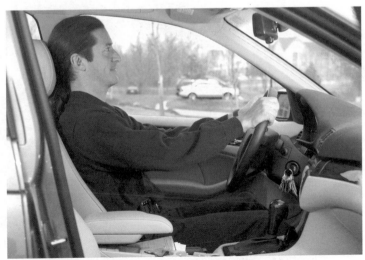

Figure 14. Person driving in car with correct posture.

- Bend at the knees and not the waist to reach for drawers that are lower to the ground (Figs. 15 and 16).

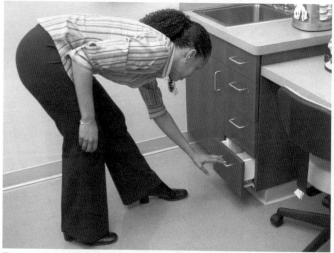

Figure 15. Person bending to open drawer with poor posture.

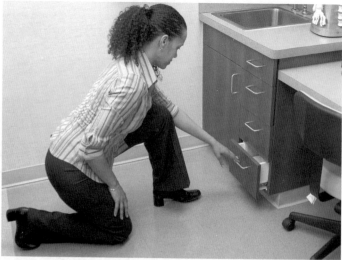

Figure 16. Person bending to open drawer with correct posture.

- While reading in bed, sit with proper lower back support (Figs. 17 and 18).

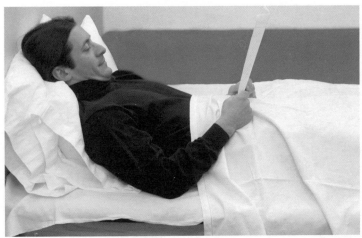

Figure 17. Person reading in a bed, slouching.

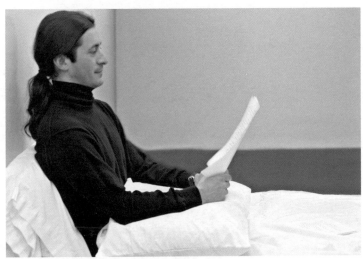

Figure 18. Person sitting in bed with proper posture.

- Avoid bending at the waist when sweeping, raking, or shoveling (Figs. 19 and 20).

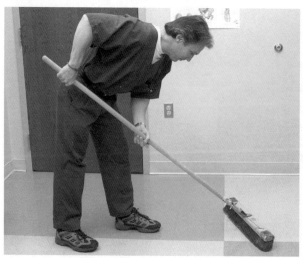

Figure 19. Person sweeping with poor posture.

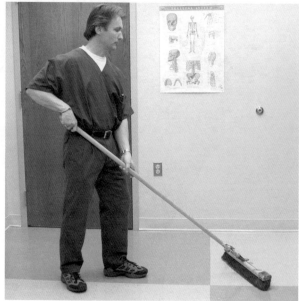

Figure 20. Person sweeping with proper posture.

- Lift objects by bending your knees, not your waist. Remember to breathe normally as you lift the object (Figs. 21 and 22).

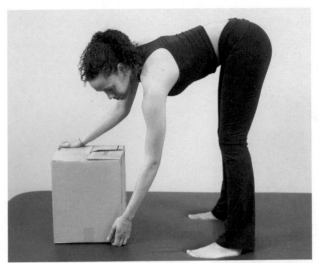

Figure 21. Bending forward with incorrect posture.

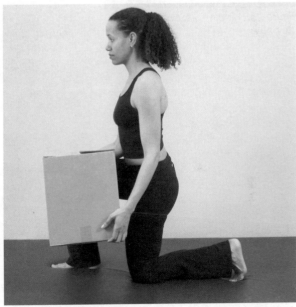

Figure 22. Lifting by squatting done/ perhaps one leg behind.

- Hold boxes close to the body to prevent excessive strain on the back muscles (Figs. 23 and 24).

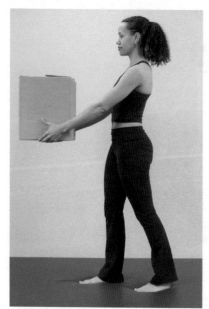

Figure 23. Holding box away from the body.

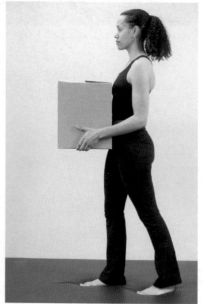

Figure 24. Holding box near body.

Treatment Options

Proper treatment of any back injury requires supervision by a physician, especially when there is trauma to the back, prolonged pain, or associated tingling involving the lower leg. Fortunately, patients have a variety of options to treat back pain symptoms. Patients should consider trying some of these basic options prior to seeking medical attention. However, patients should be sure to discuss with the physician any treatments and obtain the physician's approval before progressing with any exercises, especially if they worsen back pain.

Medication

A variety of medications may be utilized to relieve back pain symptoms and improve recovery. The most common medications are called NSAIDs or non-steroidal anti-inflammatory drugs. Common NSAIDs include ibuprofen or naproxen. These medications are helpful in treating the pain and inflammation associated with back pain. However, potential side effects include acid reflux, stomach ulcers, and problems with the kidneys. Patients should always discuss the use of any medication with a physician to assure that there are no issues preventing the use of such medications in treating pain.

Modalities and Bracing

Modalities include the application of such interventions as ice, heat, electrical stimulation, or ultrasound to the muscles of the back. Several of these modalities may be applied by the patient. Others require a licensed professional trained in its proper use.

- *Ice*: After acute injury, you should use ice for any muscle pain to reduce pain and swelling. Ice is the preferred modality to be used intermittently for the first 48 hours following an injury. Cold packs, frozen vegetable packs, or ice bags can be used. Ice packs should be wrapped in a cloth or towel so that they are not placed directly on the skin. Direct application to skin can be uncomfortable and cause damage to skin. Ice packs are most helpful if used several times a day for approximately 10 to 15 minutes.
- *Heat*: Heat helps relieve pain, and promotes circulation and muscle relaxation. Heating packs, electric heating pads, or moist heated towels can be used. Moist heat, as applied though a hot pack or warm towel,

should be applied to the involved area to help relax your muscles prior to performing gentle stretching exercises. Heat should not be used in the first 48 hours because it will increase the amount of inflammation and swelling. Heat packs should be wrapped in a cloth or towel so that they are not placed directly on the skin. Direct application to skin can be uncomfortable and burn the skin.

- *Ultrasound*: This modality utilizes heat and ultrasound waves to treat your muscle pain. Ultrasound treatment should only be applied by a professional trained in its proper use.
- *Electrical stimulation*: Electrical stimulation as applied through E-Stim or a TENS unit can assist with the reduction of pain. Similar to the use of ultrasound, the treatment should only be applied by a professional trained in its proper use.
- *Massage*: Gentle massage, consisting of kneading or stroking of the back muscles, can help alleviate some pain. However, massage is most effective when administered by a licensed professional massage therapist.
- *Back brace*: At times, some physicians will prescribe a back brace to relieve some of the stress to the muscles of your back. However, you should not use the back brace for more than a few days because prolonged use will lead to deconditioning of the back muscles and worsening pain.

Physical Therapy

For more severe pain, your physician may prescribe physical therapy to treat your back pain symptoms depending upon the cause of your pain. Physical therapists will utilize a variety of the modalities listed above to decrease your pain and increase your back's range of motion. You will then progress to a series of back stretching and strengthening exercises. These exercises are listed below and should be incorporated into a home exercise program.

Exercises

The following series of exercises is specifically designed to stretch and strengthen the muscles in your back. If you are recovering from a back strain or have chronic stiffness, you should start the exercises slowly and gradually build up your strength and endurance until you can perform them several times per day. Mild increased soreness or stiffness may occur the day after performing these exercises. However, prolonged or worsening pain should lead to an evaluation by your physician. You should discuss your exercise program with your doctor before you begin and keep your doctor informed of your progress and any problems or questions. These exercises should be incorporated into a general exercise program that includes aerobic conditioning, such as walking, running, or cycling.

Stretching

The following stretches are designed to help increase your back's range of motion. You should hold each stretch for 20 to 30 seconds and repeat each stretch two to three times, at least once a day. You should stretch the muscle until you feel a slight pull, but no further.

Exercise 1: <u>Lumbar spine stretch:</u> knees to chest. Lie flat on your back with your knees slightly bent. Very slowly bring your right knee toward your chest, while keeping your left knee bent with your left foot on the floor. You may grab the back of your right leg with your hands to further stretch the lower back. Hold the position for 20 seconds (Fig. 25). Slowly return to the starting position and repeat on the other side.

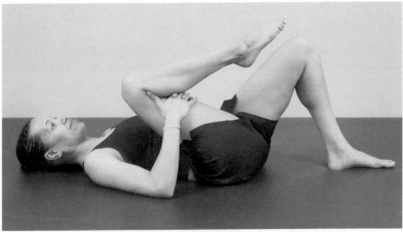

Figure 25. Lumbar stretch-supine, knees to chest.

Exercise 2: <u>Lumbar spine stretch:</u> sitting. Sit in a firm, sturdy chair. Hold your arms loosely by your sides. Lower your head toward your knees, bending at the waist. Hold the position for 20 seconds (Fig. 26). Slowly return to your starting position.

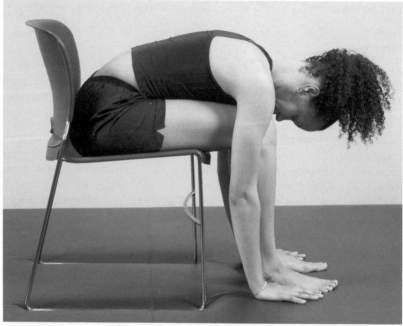

Figure 26. Lumbar stretch-sitting.

Exercise 3: <u>Lumbar spine stretch:</u> knees to side. Lie flat on your back with your knees bent (Fig. 27a). Slowly bend your legs and hips to the left. You may place your left hand on the top of your right knee to assist with the stretch. Hold the position for 20 seconds. Slowly return to your starting position. Repeat to the opposite side.

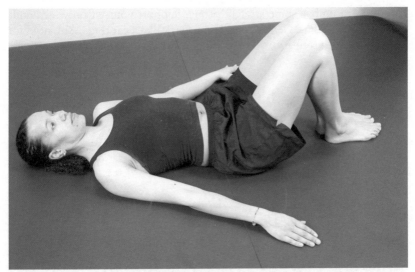

Figure 27a. Lumbar stretch-supine, knees to side-start position.

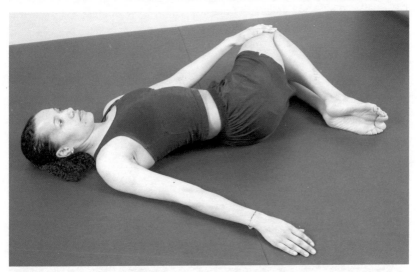

Figure 27b. Lumbar stretch-supine, knees to side-exercise.

Exercise 4: <u>Lumbar spine stretch:</u> prone. Support yourself on your hands and knees (Fig. 28a). Gently round your back like a cat (Fig. 28b), hold for 20 seconds, and return to your starting position.

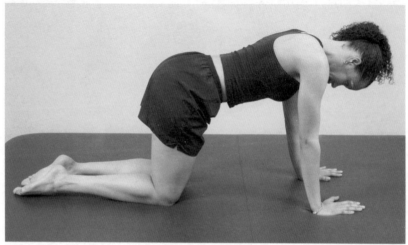

Figure 28a. Cat lumbar stretch-start position.

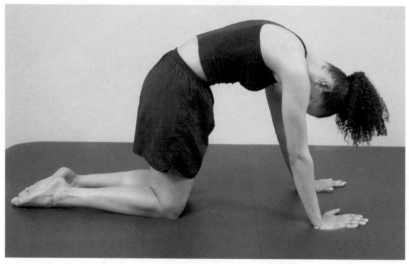

Figure 28b. Cat lumbar stretch-exercise.

Exercise 5: <u>Hamstring stretch:</u> sitting. Sit on the floor with your legs closed in front of you. Gently lean forward with your chest, keeping your lower back straight until you feel a pull in the hamstring region (Fig. 29). Keep your knees straight.

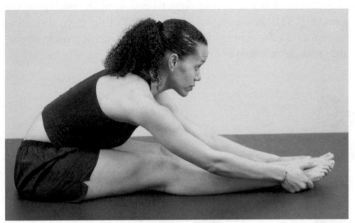

Figure 29. Hamstring stretch, sitting.

Exercise 6: <u>Hip Flexor Stretch:</u> (Caution: perform this exercise on a mat to minimize any knee discomfort.) Start with your weight on your right knee and left foot. Gently lean forward with your left knee to produce a stretch in the front of the right hip (Fig. 30). Make sure to keep your left knee directly above your ankle, not forward over your toes. Return to your starting position and repeat on the other side.

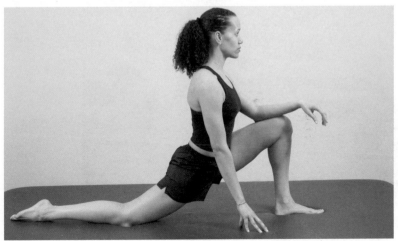

Figure 30. Hip flexor stretch.

Exercise 7: Quadriceps Stretch: Start by standing with both feet together and your hands by your sides. While standing on your left leg, grab your right foot on the opposite leg with your right hand and pull the foot toward the buttock region until you feel a pull in your thigh (Fig. 31a). Remember to keep your pelvis level and your foot toward the middle of the buttock region (Fig. 31b shows incorrect position). Return to your starting position and repeat on the other side. If this is too difficult, you may perform the same maneuver while lying on your stomach (Fig. 31c).

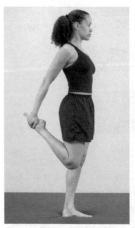 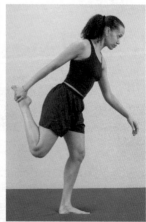

Figure 31a. CORRECT.   *Figure 31c.* INCORRECT.

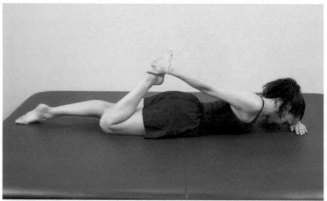

Figure 31c. CORRECT. Quad stretch, standing and lying.

Strengthening

After your pain has decreased and your range of motion has improved, you may gradually start your strengthening exercise program. These back exercises are designed to increase your overall strength and stamina. You should hold each position for approximately 3 to 5 seconds and relax. Repeat each exercise three to five times as tolerated. Be sure to breathe properly throughout the exercises.

Exercise 1: <u>Pelvic Tilts.</u> Lie on your back with your knees bent (Fig. 32a). Gently pull your navel toward the floor as your pelvis slowly rotates up from the bottom (Fig. 32b). Hold the position for 3 to 5 seconds and return to the starting position. Repeat three to five times.

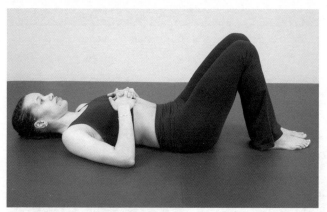

Figure 32a. Pelvic tilts-start.

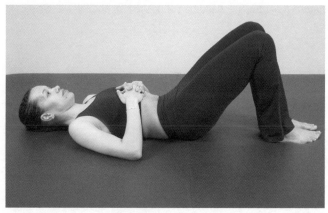

Figure 32b. Pelvic tilts-exercise.

Exercise 2: <u>Dead Bug.</u> Lie on your back with your legs flat on the ground and your left arm over your head (Fig. 33a). Gently lift your right leg and left arm several inches off the floor (Fig. 33b). Hold the position for 2 to 5 seconds and return to the starting position. Repeat three to five times and on the opposite side.

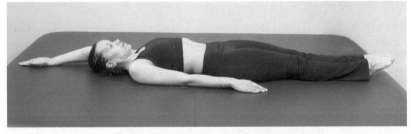

Figure 33a. Supine, dead bug opposite arm and leg-start position.

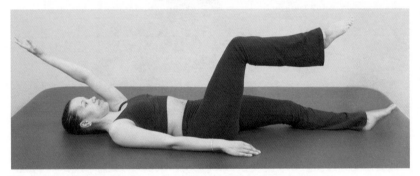

Figure 33b. Supine, dead bug opposite arm and leg-exercise.

Exercise 3: <u>Superman.</u> Start on your hands and knees with a flat back (Fig. 34a). Gently lift your right leg and left arm until they are in line with your spine (Fig. 34b). Hold the position for 3 to 5 seconds and return to the starting position. Repeat on the opposite side.

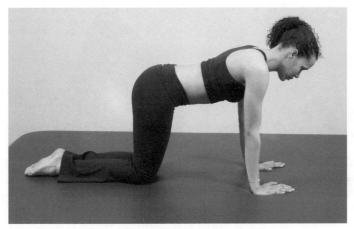

Figure 34a. Prone, opposite arm and leg-start position.

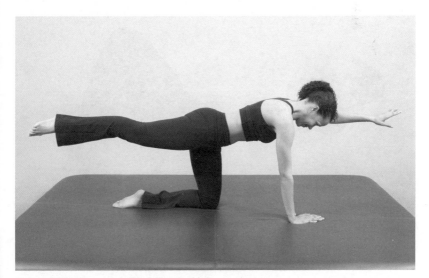

Figure 34b. Prone, opposite arm and leg-exercise.

Exercise 4: <u>Abdominal Exercises.</u> Lie on your back with your knees bent and hands behind your head or crossed on your chest (Fig. 35a). Gently lift your head and upper torso several inches off the floor by tightening your abdominal muscles (Fig. 35b). Hold the position for 2 to 5 seconds and return to the starting position.

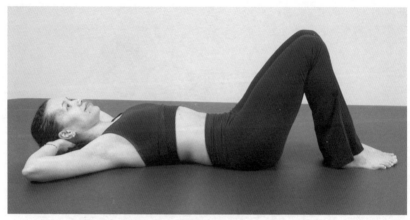

Figure 35a. Abdominal exercise-start position.

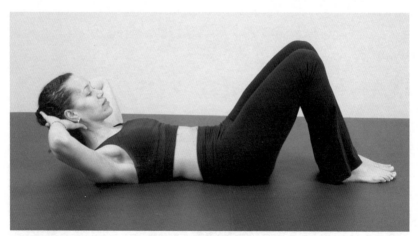

Figure 35b. Abdominal exercise.

Summary

1. Back pain is often due to muscle strains, which can be treated by proper rest, activity modification, medication, and exercises to improve posture. Severe back pain or stiffness that does not respond to the above interventions could indicate a more serious problem that requires medical attention.

2. Attempt to avoid the habit of sitting with the head thrust too far forward and back hunched over. Learn to stand and sit properly. This is especially important if a job puts the patient in a position that causes strain to the back for a prolonged period of time.

3. Do not slump or slouch in unnatural positions while performing daily activities.

4. The patient should be sure to get enough rest. Stress and tiredness can contribute to back pain symptoms.

5. Exercise to stretch and strengthen the muscles in the back. The patient should perform these exercises several times per week to maintain proper flexibility and strength.

6. The patient should incorporate back exercises into a generalized exercise program including aerobic conditioning.

Notes